REFLEX TESTING METHODS
for
EVALUATING C.N.S. DEVELOPMENT

Publication Number 865

AMERICAN LECTURE SERIES®

A Monograph in

AMERICAN LECTURES IN ORTHOPAEDIC SURGERY

Edited by

CHARLES WEER GOFF, M.D.

*Associate Clinical Professor of Orthopaedics
and Lecturer in Anatomy
Yale University, School of Medicine
Hartford, Connecticut*

REFLEX TESTING METHODS
for
EVALUATING C.N.S. DEVELOPMENT

Second Edition

By

MARY R. FIORENTINO, MUS. B., O.T.R.

Director of Occupational Therapy
Newington Children's Hospital
Newington, Connecticut

With a Foreword by
Burr H. Curtis, M.D.
Medical Director
Newington Children's Hospital
Newington, Connecticut

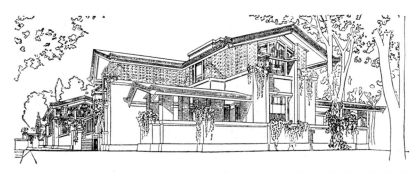

CHARLES C THOMAS • PUBLISHER
Springfield • *Illinois* • *U.S.A.*

Published and Distributed Throughout the World by
CHARLES C THOMAS • PUBLISHER

BANNERSTONE HOUSE
301-327 East Lawrence Avenue, Springfield, Illinois, U.S.A.

© *1963 and 1973,* CHARLES C THOMAS • PUBLISHER
ISBN 0-398-02584-3
Library of Congress Catalog Card Number: 72-86999

First Edition, First Printing, 1963
First Edition, Second Printing, 1965
First Edition, Third Printing, 1968
First Edition, Fourth Printing, 1969
First Edition, Fifth Printing, 1970
First Edition, Sixth Printing, 1971
Second Edition, First Printing, 1973

Printed in the United States of America
HH-11

This manual is dedicated to the therapists in my department for their conscientious and diligent cooperation in the application of a method of treatment that has been found effective for the child with cerebral palsy.

FOREWORD

IN THE development of the program for the cerebrally handicapped at Newington Children's Hospital, the necessity for an increasing awareness of what is normal has prompted Miss Fiorentino and others to better document the normal reflex development in children.

Miss Fiorentino has accomplished this through considerable personal effort. She is gifted with a rare ability to impart this information to physicians, other therapists and students. Requests for her knowledge of the subject led her to the writing of this manual which should provide a better understanding of the reflex patterns of both normal children and those afflicted with neurological disorders, and should aid medical and paramedical persons dealing with such children in establishment of diagnosis, programming and recording of progress in their habilitation.

BURR H. CURTIS, M.D.
Medical Director
Newington Children's Hospital
Newington, Connecticut

PREFACE

IT IS believed that a clearer understanding of normal, neurophysiological development and methods of testing will be helpful to physicians and paramedical personnel working closely with handicapped children. It is hoped that this will assist in the evaluation, diagnosis and assessment of children through six years of age, and in programming rehabilitation of neurophysiologically involved children. The testing methods will be of value to the following:

Pediatricians

In the initial and periodic examination of all infants and children through six years of age.

Neurologists

In the diagnosis and evaluation of infants and children where abnormal reflexive reactions are suspected.

Orthopaedists

For the assessment of patients who would lend themselves to a neurophysiologically oriented treatment.

Physiatrists

A basis for diagnosis and program-planning for rehabilitation.

Occupational, Physical and Speech Therapists

To determine the maturational level and abnormal reflexes for a treatment program.

ACKNOWLEDGMENTS

GRATEFUL appreciation is extended to Edward D. Mysak, Ph.D., former speech pathologist at Newington Children's Hospital, for introducing this method to the Hospital and this department, and without whose guidance and teaching in the basic theories of the Neurophysiological Approach, this manual would not have been possible at this time.

To the following members of the staff of the Newington Children's Hospital for their assistance and cooperation in making this manual possible: Burr H. Curtis, M.D., Medical Director; John C. Allen, M.D., Visiting Physiatrist; Otto G. Goldkamp, M.D., Associate Physiatrist; Walter F. Jennings, M.D., Myron E. Shafer, M.D., and Charles W. Goff, M.D., members of the orthopaedic staff; Miss Carol Nathan, O.T.R., Assistant Director of Occupational Therapy; Miss Ann P. Grady, O.T.R., staff therapist; Mr. William McCarthy, high school teacher; the photography department; the children and their parents who allowed their pictures to be used.

To Associate Professor Frieda J. Behlen, M.A., O.T.R., Advisor, Occupational Therapy Curriculum, New York University, for her sincere efforts and interest in this manual.

To Barry S. Russman, M.D., staff Pediatric Neurologist, and Miss Constance M. Lundberg, O.T.R., Student Supervisor, for their assistance in the revision of this book.

Photographs taken by Miss Carol Nathan, O.T.R.

M.R.F.

CONTENTS

REFLEX TESTING METHODS
for
EVALUATING C.N.S. DEVELOPMENT

INTRODUCTION

EARLY diagnosis of persistent abnormal reflexes may be of great significance to a more effective functioning of the cerebral palsied child. We feel that knowledge of normal and abnormal reflex responses and their effect upon motor development is needed to provide a basis for evaluation in the diagnosis and treatment of the cerebral palsied child and certain other cerebral dysfunctions.

Since Little applied the term "spastic paralysis" to all cerebral palsied children in 1843, much research has been undertaken in an attempt to understand the physical, mental, perceptual, visual, auditory, epileptic and psycho-social manifestations of neurological dysfunctions. Though scientist and clinician have contributed much to our knowledge, there is need for further investigation in both theory and therapy of C.N.S. abnormalities.

Some of the recent advances in this country are based upon knowledge of the neurophysiological implication of reflexive maturation of the C.N.S. The rationale of treatment and therapeutic application of this approach was described by the Bobaths *et al.* Knowledge gained from this approach can be applied to testing and evaluating the normal, sequential growth and maturation of any child.

PURPOSE

THE purpose of this manual is to orient the physicians and the various paramedical disciplines to a method of evaluating C.N.S. dysfunction utilizing neurophysiological principles. To accomplish its goal, the manual presents the following:

1. Normal sequential development of reflexive maturation.

2. Possible abnormal responses found in individuals with C.N.S. disorders, such as cerebral palsy.

3. Reflex Testing and Motor Development Charts to assist in the rating of normal and abnormal responses (see pages 50-52).

Purpose of Testing

To determine neurophysiological reflexive maturation of the C.N.S. at the spinal, brain stem, midbrain and cortical levels. This maturation has been determined in animals, as described by Sherrington. We feel that we can assume similar reflexes seen in humans might correlate in their pattern of neurological maturation.

Who Should Test

Tests are designed for all those evaluating and treating children with neurophysiological dysfunctions, namely, the general practitioner, pediatrician, neurologist, orthopaedist, physiatrist, occupational, physical and speech therapists.

When to Test

The initial and periodic examination of all children from infancy, of full-term gestation, through the age of six years, as well as older children demonstrating abnormal reflexes. Therapy should begin before children develop abnormal patterns of turning, sitting, crawling and walking. *Early referral* of patients for reflex therapy cannot be over-emphasized.

RATIONALE

WE feel that primitive reflexes are essential in normal development. Response to these reflexes prepares the child for progressive development, such as rolling over, sitting, crawling, standing, etc. It is to be understood that a child may omit one level of development, such as creeping, and still continue the normal process of developmental maturation. In normal development, these primitive spinal and brain stem reflexes gradually diminish in order that higher patterns of righting and equilibrium reactions may become manifested. When inhibitory control of higher centers is disrupted or delayed, primitive patterns dominate to the exclusion of higher, integrated sensorimotor activities. Certain neurologic dysfunctions are believed to result from specific C.N.S. lesions. Such lesions release primitive, abnormal reflexes from inhibition normally exerted by higher centers. These more primitive reflexes result in abnormalities manifested by phylogenetically older postures and movements and abnormal muscle tone, as seen in cerebral palsied children.

Following the above concept, the cerebral palsied child can be classified according to sequential development of reflex maturation and evaluated in terms of the status of his particular level of reflexology and abnormal muscle tone. There are three levels of reflexive development:

Apedal—predominance of primitive spinal and brain stem reflexes with motor development of a prone or supine-lying creature.

Quadrupedal—predominance of midbrain development with righting reactions and motor development that of a child who can right himself, turn over, assume crawling and sitting positions.

Bipedal—at cortical level of development reveals equilibrium reactions,

TABLE I
NORMAL SEQUENTIAL DEVELOPMENT

Levels of C.N.S. Maturation	Corresponding Levels of Reflexive Development	Resulting Levels of Motor Development
Spinal and/or Brain Stem	Apedal Primitive Reflexes	Prone-lying Supine-lying
Midbrain	Quadrupedal Righting Reactions	Crawling Sitting
Cortical	Bipedal Equilibrium Reactions	Standing Walking

with motor development that of a child who can assume the standing position and ambulate.

In neurologic dysfunction, varying degrees and combinations of the above levels may be seen in any one child. Knowledge of normal and abnormal reflex responses and their effect on motor behavior will aid in better understanding the nature of the neurophysiologic dysfunction, and in providing a basis for evaluation.

PROCEDURE

THE following pages present photographs and explanation of the four levels of the C.N.S. in their sequence of reflexive maturation. Photographs and explanations of reflex responses within the four levels and test positions with normal and abnormal responses are illustrated. *Negative reactions* of the first two levels imply *normal* responses; *positive reactions, abnormal responses. Negative reactions* of the upper two levels imply *abnormal* responses; *positive reactions, normal* responses. Each reflex tested can be rated on a Reflex Testing Chart and resulting functional responses on a Motor Development Chart.

These reflexes are normal within certain age limits and should be interpreted as abnormal beyond those limits. Normal growth and developmental levels vary somewhat; therefore, *age levels* are *approximate.*

SPINAL LEVEL

SPINAL reflexes are mediated by areas of the C.N.S. Deiters' nucleus which is in the lower third of the pons.

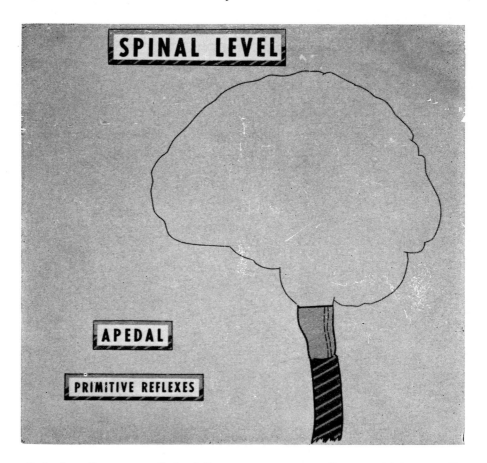

Spinal reflexes are "phasic" or movement reflexes which coordinate muscles of the extremities in patterns of either total flexion or extension. Positive or negative reactions to spinal reflex testing may be present in the normal child within the first two months of life. Positive reactions persisting beyond two months of age may be indicative of delayed maturation of the C.N.S. Negative reactions are normal. Complete domination by these primitive spinal reflexes results in an apedal (prone, supine-lying) creature.

Flexor Withdrawal   Extensor Thrust   Crossed Extension

Flexor Withdrawal

Negative Reaction

Test Position

Patient supine.
Head in mid-position.
Legs extended.

Test Stimulus

Stimulate sole of foot.

Negative Reaction

Controlled maintenance of stimulated leg in extension or volitional withdrawal from irritating stimulus.

Positive Reaction

Uncontrolled flexion response of stimulated leg. (Do not confuse with response to tickling.)

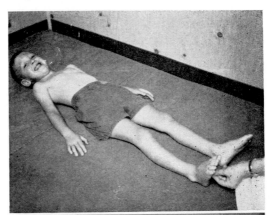

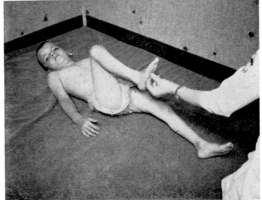

Positive Reaction

Positive reaction is normal up to two months of age. Positive reaction after two months of age may be one indication of delayed reflexive maturation.

Extensor Thrust

Negative Reaction

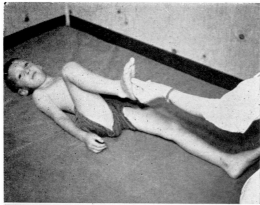

Test Position

> Patient supine.
> Head in mid-position.
> One leg extended, opposite leg flexed.

Test Stimulus

> Stimulate sole of foot of flexed leg.

Negative Reaction

> Controlled maintenance of leg in flexion.

Positive Reaction

> Uncontrolled extension of stimulated leg. (Do not confuse with response to tickling.)

Positive Reaction

Positive reaction is normal up to two months of age. Positive reaction after two months of age may be one indication of delayed reflexive maturation.

Crossed Extension

Negative Reaction

Test Position

Patient supine.
Head in mid-position.
One leg flexed, opposite leg
extended.

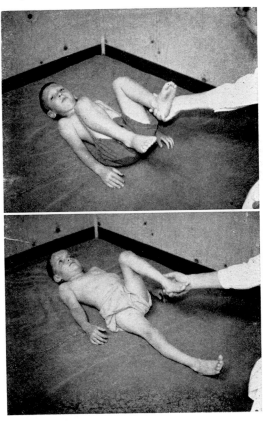

Test Stimulus

Flex the extended leg.

Negative Reaction

On flexion of the extended leg,
the opposite leg will remain
flexed.

Positive Reaction

On flexion of the extended leg,
the opposite, or initially
flexed, leg will extend.

Positive Reaction

Positive reaction is normal up to two months of age. Positive reaction after
two months of age may be one indication of delayed reflexive maturation.

Crossed Extension

Negative Reaction

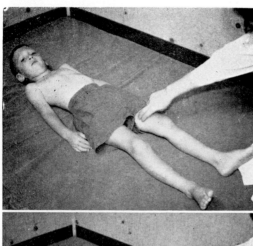

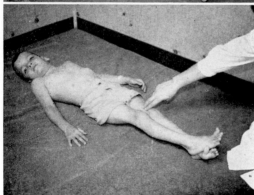

Positive Reaction

Test Position

> Patient supine.
> Head in mid-position.
> Legs extended.

Test Stimulus

> Stimulate the medial surface
> of one leg by tapping.

Negative Reaction

> No reaction of either leg
> upon stimulation.

Positive Reaction

> Opposite leg adducts,
> internally rotates and foot
> plantar flexes. (Typical
> scissor position.)

Positive reaction is normal up to two months of age. Positive reaction after two months of age may be one indication of delayed reflexive maturation.

BRAIN STEM LEVEL

B RAIN stem reflexes are mediated by areas from Deiters' nucleus to the red nucleus which sits at the most caudal level of the basal ganglia.

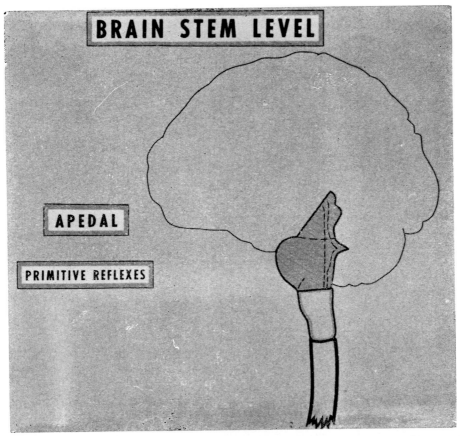

Brain stem reflexes are "static" postural reflexes and effect changes in distribution of muscle tone throughout the body, either in response to a change of the position of head and body in space (by stimulation of the labyrinths), or in the head in relation to the body (by stimulation of proprioceptors of the neck muscles). Positive or negative reactions to brain stem reflex testing may be present in the normal child within the first four to six months of life. Positive reactions persisting beyond six months of age may be indicative of delayed motor maturation of the C.N.S. Negative reactions are normal. Complete domination by these primitive brain stem reflexes results in an apedal (prone, supine-lying) creature.

Asymmetrical Tonic Neck   Symmetrical Tonic Neck
Tonic Labyrinthine—Supine Tonic Labythine—Prone Associated Reactions
Positive Supporting Reaction   Negative Supporting Reaction

Asymmetrical Tonic Neck

Negative Reaction

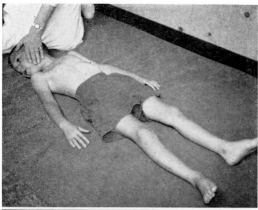

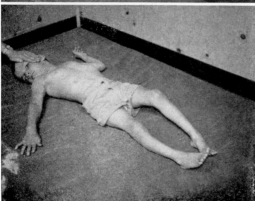

Positive Reaction

Test Position

Patient supine.
Head in mid-position.
Arms and legs extended.

Test Stimulus

Turn head to one side.

Negative Reaction

No reaction of limbs on
either side.

Positive Reaction

Extension of arm and leg on
face side, or increase in
extensor tone; flexion of
arm and leg on skull side, or
increase in flexor tone.

Positive reaction is normal up to four to six months of age. An obligatory ASTN reflex is pathologic at any age. Positive reactions after six months of age may be one indication of delayed reflexive maturation.

Symmetrical Tonic Neck 1

Negative Reaction

Test Position

Patient in quadruped position or over tester's knees.

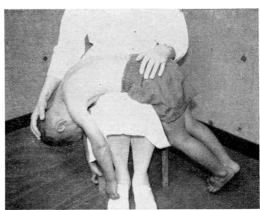

Test Stimulus

Ventroflex the head.

Negative Reaction

No change in tone of arms or legs.

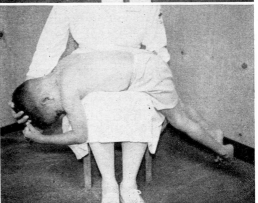

Positive Reaction

Arms flex or flexor tone dominates; legs extended or extensor tone dominates.

Positive Reaction

Positive reaction is normal up to four to six months of age. Positive reaction after six months of age may be one indication of delayed reflexive maturation.

Symmetrical Tonic Neck 2

Negative Reaction

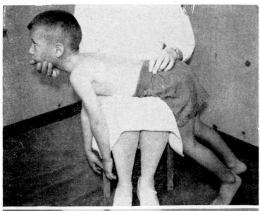

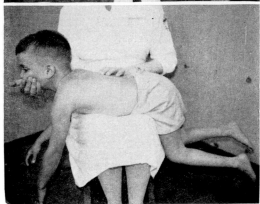

Positive Reaction

Test Position

Patient in quadruped position or over tester's knees.

Test Stimulus

Dorsiflex the head.

Negative Reaction

No change in tone of arms or legs.

Positive Reaction

Arms extend or extensor tone dominates; legs flex or flexor tone dominates.

Positive reaction is normal up to four to six months of age. Positive reaction after six months of age may be one indication of delayed reflexive maturation.

Tonic Labyrinthine Supine

Test Position

Patient supine.
Head in mid-position.
Arms and legs extended.

Test Stimulus

The supine position, per se.

Negative Reaction

No increase in extensor tone
when arms and legs are
passively flexed.

Positive Reaction

Extensor tone dominates when
arms and legs are passively
flexed.

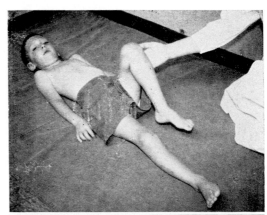

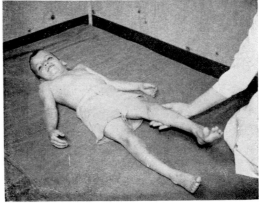

Positive Reaction

Positive reaction is normal up to four months of age. Positive reaction after four months of age may be one indication of delayed reflexive maturation.

Tonic Labyrinthine Prone

Negative Reaction

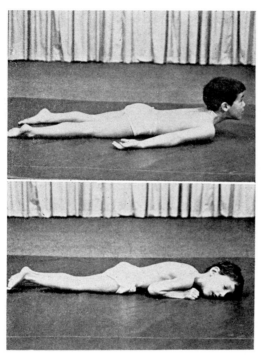

Positive Reaction

Test Position

Turn patient prone.
Head in mid-position.

Test Stimulus

Prone position, per se.

Negative Reaction

No increase in flexor tone;
head, trunk, arms, legs
can be extended.

Positive Reaction

Unable to dorsiflex head,
retract shoulders, extend
trunk, arms, legs.

Positive reaction is normal up to four months of age. Positive reaction after four months of age may be one indication of delayed reflexive maturation.

Associated Reactions

Negative Reaction

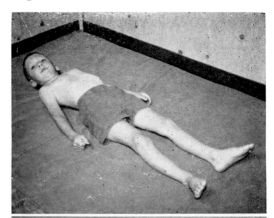

Test Position

Patient supine.

Test Stimulus

Have patient squeeze an object. (With a hemiplegic, squeeze with uninvolved hand.)

Negative Reaction

No reaction, or minimal reaction or increase of tone in other parts of the body.

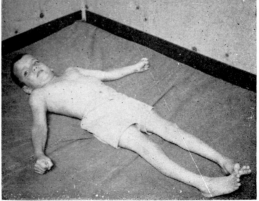

Positive Reaction

Mirroring of opposite limb and/or increase of tone in other parts of the body.

Positive Reaction

Positive reaction in patients with other abnormal reflexology may be an indication of delayed reflexive maturation.

Negative Reaction

Positive Supporting Reaction

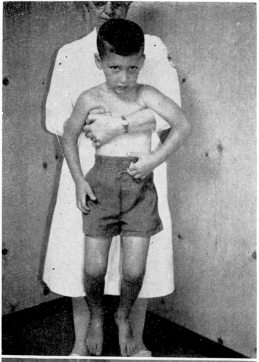

Test Position

Hold patient in standing position.

Test Stimulus

Bounce several times on soles of feet.

Negative Reaction

No increase of tone (legs volitionally flex).

Positive Reaction

Increase of extensor tone in legs. Plantar flexion of feet, genu recurvatum may occur.

Positive reaction is normal from three to eight months of age. Positive reaction after eight months of age may be one indication of delayed reflexive maturation.

Positive Reaction

Negative Supporting Reaction

Test Position

Bring patient to standing position.

Test Stimulus

Weight-bearing position.

Negative Reaction

Release of extensor tone from positive supporting allows plantigrade feet and flexion of legs.

Positive Reaction

No release of extensor tone, positive supporting persists.

Normal reaction is sufficient release of extensor tone to allow flexion for reciprocation. Abnormal reaction is continuation of positive supporting reflex beyond eight months of age. A reaction of excessive flexion on weight bearing is abnormal beyond four months of age.

Negative Reaction

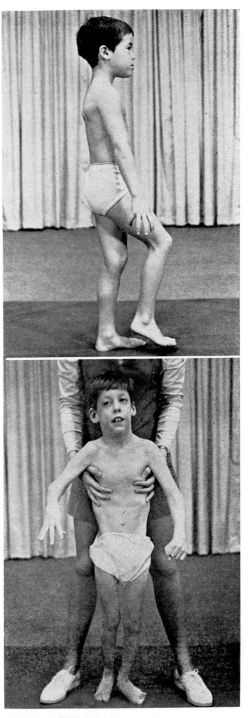

Positive Reaction

MIDBRAIN LEVEL

Righting reactions are integrated at the midbrain level above the red nucleus, not including the cortex.

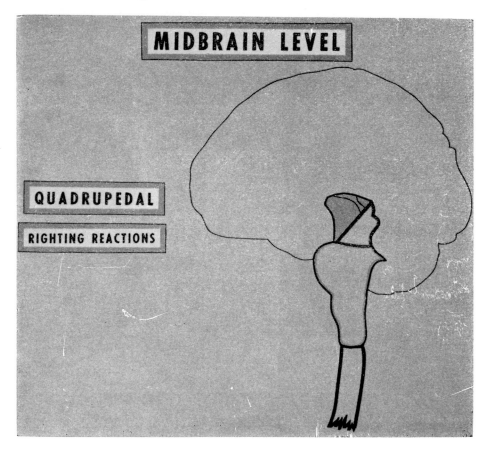

Righting reactions interact with each other and work toward establishment of normal head and body relationship in space as well as in relation to each other. These are the first such reactions to develop after birth and reach maximal concerted effect about age ten to twelve months. As cortical control increases, they are gradually modified and inhibited and disappear towards the end of the fifth year. Their combined actions enable the child to roll over, sit up, get on his hands and knees, and make him a quadrupedal creature.

Neck Righting   Body Righting Acting on the Body
Labyrinthine Righting Acting on the Head   Optical Righting Acting on the
Head Amphibian

Neck Righting

Test Position

Patient supine.
Head in mid-position.
Arms and legs extended.

Test Stimulus

Rotate head to one side,
actively or passively.

Negative Reaction

Body will not rotate.

Positive Reaction

Body rotates as a whole in the
same direction as the head.

Positive reaction is normal
from birth to six months of
age. Positive reaction beyond
six months of age may be one
indication of delayed reflexive
maturation. Negative reaction
over one month of age is one
indication of delayed reflexive
maturation.

Negative Reaction

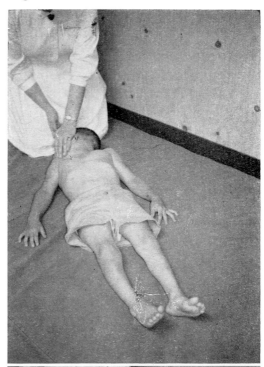

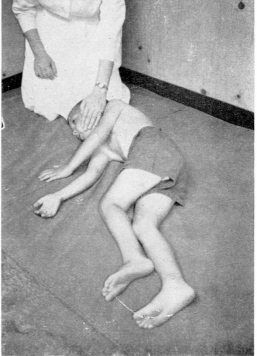

Positive Reaction

Body Righting Acting on the Body

Negative Reaction

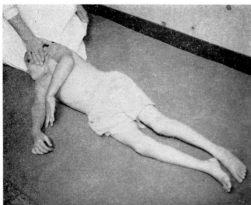

Test Position

Patient supine.
Head in mid-position.
Arms and legs extended.

Test Stimulus

Rotate head to one side,
actively or passively.

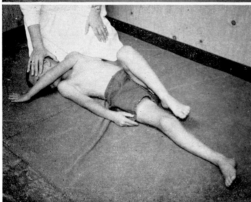

Negative Reaction

Body rotates as a whole
(neck righting), and not
segmentally.

Positive Reaction

Segmental rotation of trunk
between shoulders and pelvis,
e.g. head turns, then
shoulders, finally the pelvis.

Positive Reaction

Positive reaction emerges about six months of age and continues to eighteen months of age. Negative reaction over six months of age may be one indication of delayed reflexive maturation.

Labyrinthine Righting Acting on the Head 1

Negative Reaction

Test Position

Hold blindfolded patient in space.
Prone position.

Test Stimulus

Prone position in space, per se.

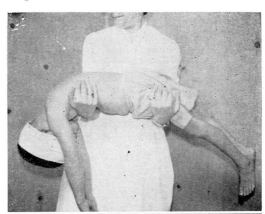

Negative Reaction

Head does not raise automatically to the normal position.

Positive Reaction

Head raises to normal position, face vertical, mouth horizontal.

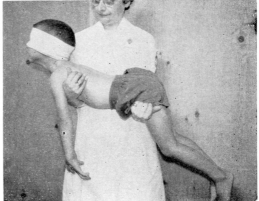

Positive Reaction

Positive reaction is normal about one to two months of age and continues throughout life. Negative reaction after two months of age may be one indication of delayed reflexive maturation.

Labyrinthine Righting Acting on the Head 2

Negative Reaction

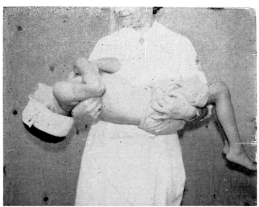

Test Position

Hold blindfolded patient
in space.
Supine position.

Test Stimulus

Supine position in space,
per se.

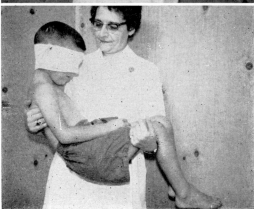

Negative Reaction

Head does not raise
automatically to the
normal position.

Positive Reaction

Head raises to normal
position, face vertical,
mouth horizontal.

Positive Reaction

Positive reaction is normal about six months of age and continues
throughout life. Negative reaction after six months of age may be one
indication of delayed reflexive maturation.

Labyrinthine Righting Acting on the Head 3

Negative Reaction

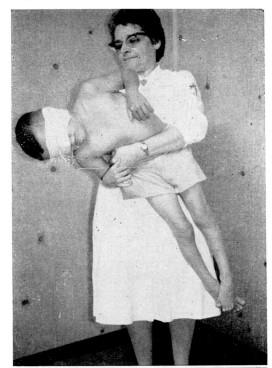

Test Position

Hold blindfolded patient in space.
Hold around pelvis.

Test Stimulus

Tilt to the right.

Negative Reaction

Head does not right itself automatically to the normal position.

Positive Reaction

Head rights itself to normal position, face vertical, mouth horizontal.

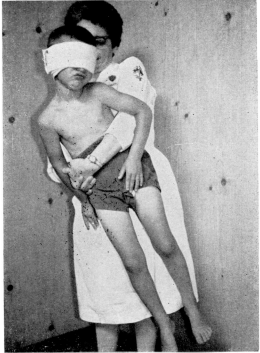

Positive reaction is normal about six to eight months of age and continues throughout life. Negative reaction after eight months of age may be one indication of delayed reflexive maturation.

Positive Reaction

Negative Reaction

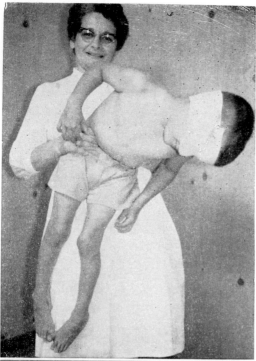

Labyrinthine Righting Acting on the Head 4

Test Position

Hold blindfolded patient in space.
Hold around pelvis.

Test Stimulus

Tilt to the left.

Negative Reaction

Head does not right itself automatically to the normal position.

Positive Reaction

Head rights itself to normal position, face vertical, mouth horizontal.

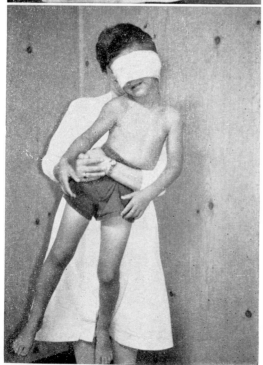

Positive Reaction

Positive reaction is normal about six to eight months of age and continues throughout life. Negative reaction after eight months of age may be one indication of delayed reflexive maturation.

Optical Righting 1

Negative Reaction

Test Position

Hold patient in space.
Prone position.

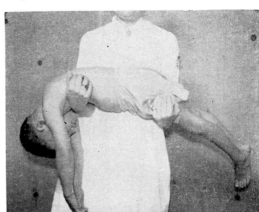

Test Stimulus

Prone position in space,
per se.

Negative Reaction

Head does not raise
automatically to the
normal position.

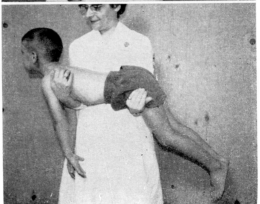

Positive Reaction

Head raises to normal
position, face vertical,
mouth horizontal.

Positive Reaction

Positive reaction normally appears soon after labyrinthine righting acting on the head (1-2 months) and continues throughout life. (Optical righting reactions in all positions are valid only if the labyrinthine righting is not present). Negative reaction after this time may be one indication of delayed reflexive maturation.

Optical Righting 2

Negative Reaction

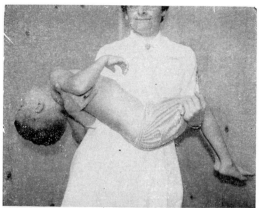

Positive Reaction

Test Position

Hold patient in space.
Supine position.

Test Stimulus

Supine position in space,
per se.

Negative Reaction

Head does not raise
automatically to the
normal position.

Positive Reaction

Head raises to normal
position, face vertical,
mouth horizontal.

Positive reaction is normal about six months of age and continues
throughout life. Negative reaction after six months of age may be one indication of delayed reflexive maturation.

Optical Righting 3

Negative Reaction

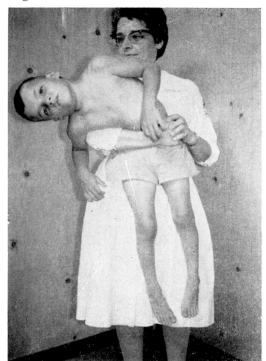

Test Position

Hold patient in space.
Hold around pelvis.

Test Stimulus

Tilt to the right.

Negative Reaction

Head does not right itself
automatically to the
normal position.

Positive Reaction

Head rights itself to normal
position, face vertical,
mouth horizontal.

Positive reaction is normal
about six to eight months of
age and continues throughout
life. Negative reaction after
eight months of age may be
one indication of delayed reflexive maturation.

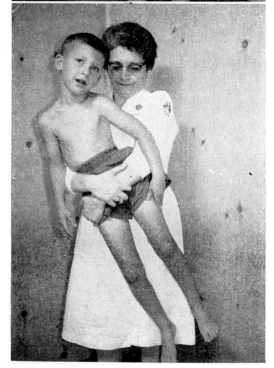

Positive Reaction

Negative Reaction   **Optical Righting 4**

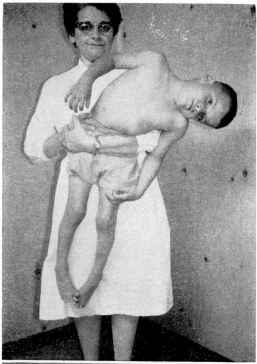

Test Position

Hold patient in space.
Hold around pelvis.

Test Stimulus

Tilt to the left.

Negative Reaction

Head does not right
itself automatically to
the normal position.

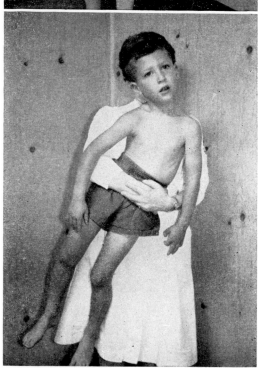

Positive Reaction

Head rights itself to normal
position, face vertical,
mouth horizontal.

Positive reaction is normal
about six to eight months of
age and continues throughout
life. Negative reaction after
eight months of age may be
one indication of delayed reflexive maturation.

Positive Reaction

Amphibian Reaction

Negative Reaction

Test Position

> Patient prone.
> Head in mid-position.
> Legs extended, arms
> extended over head.

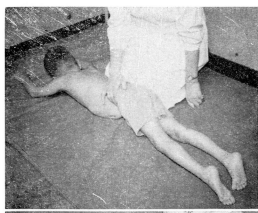

Test Stimulus

> Lift pelvis on one side.

Negative Reaction

> Flexion of arm, hip and knee
> cannot be elicited.

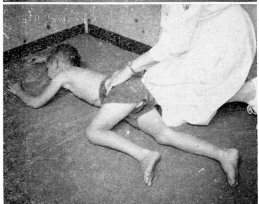

Positive Reaction

> Automatic flexion of arm,
> hip and knee on same side.

Positive Reaction

Positive reaction is normal at six months of age and remains throughout life. Negative reaction after six months of age may be one indication of delayed reflexive maturation.

AUTOMATIC MOVEMENT REACTIONS

T HESE are described as a group of reflexes observed in infants and young children which are not strictly righting reflexes, but which are reactions produced by changes in the position of the head and, hypothetically, involve either the semicircular canals, or labyrinths, or neck proprioceptors. Like righting reflexes, they appear at certain stages of development and their persistence, or absence, can be observed in patients under pathological conditions.

Moro Reflex   Landau Reflex   Protective Extensor Thrust

Moro Reflex

Negative Reaction

Test Position

Patient in semi-reclined position.

Test Stimulus

Drop head backward.

Negative Reaction

Minimal or no startle response.

Positive Reaction

Abduction, extension (or flexion), external rotation of arms; extension and abduction of the fingers.

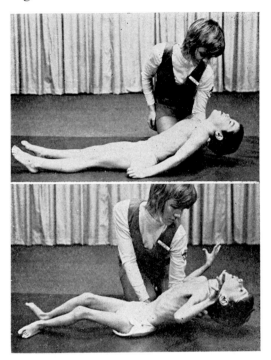

Positive Reaction

Positive reaction is normal from birth to four months of age. Positive reaction after four months of age may be one indication of delayed reflexive maturation. Negative reaction is normal after four months of age.

Landau Reflex

Negative Reaction

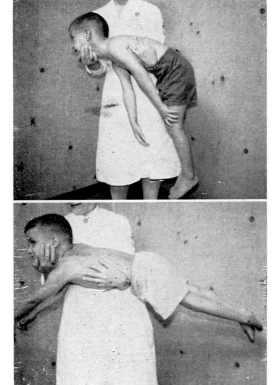

Positive Reaction

Test Position

Patient held in space,
supporting thorax.
Prone position.

Test Stimulus

Head raised, actively
or passively.

Negative Reaction

Spine and legs remain in
flexed position

Positive Reaction

Spine and legs extend.
(When head is ventroflexed,
spine and legs flex.)

Positive reaction is normal from six months to two or two and one half years of age. Positive reaction after two and one half years of age may be one indication of delayed reflexive maturation. Negative reaction is normal from birth to six months of age and from two and one half years through out life.

Protective Extensor Thrust (Parachute Reaction)

Negative Reaction

Test Position

Patient prone.
Arms extended overhead.

Test Stimulus

Suspend patient in air by
ankles or pelvis and move
head suddenly towards floor.

Negative Reaction

Arms do not protect head, but
show primitive reflex reaction,
such as, asymmetrical or
symmetrical tonic neck
reflexes.

Positive Reaction

Immediate extension of arms
with abduction and extension
of fingers to protect the head.

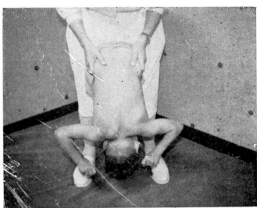

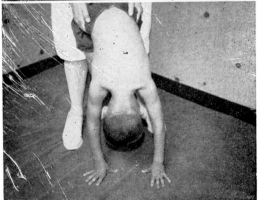

Positive Reaction

Positive reaction is normal about six months of age and remains throughout life. Negative reaction after six months of age may be one indication
of delayed reflexive maturation.

CORTICAL LEVEL

THESE reactions are mediated by the efficient interaction of cortex, basal ganglia and cerebellum.

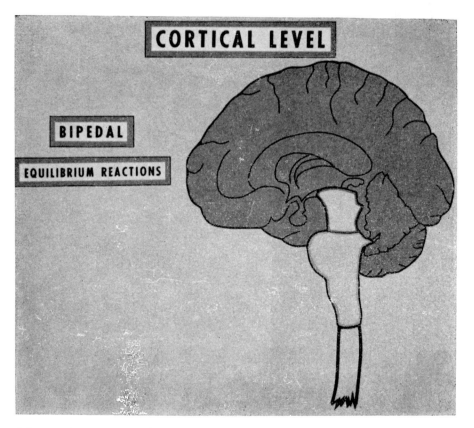

Maturation of equilibrium reactions brings the individual to the human bipedal stage of motor development. They occur when muscle tone is normalized and provide body adaptation in response to change of center of gravity in the body. They emerge from six months on. Positive reaction at any one level indicates the next higher level of motor activity is possible.

Supine   Prone   Four-Foot Kneeling   Sitting   Kneel-Standing
Standing-Hopping   Doriflexion   See-Saw   Simian Position

Supine

Negative Reaction

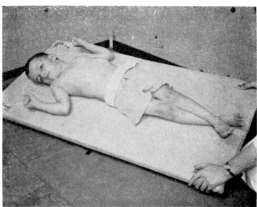

Test Position

Patient supine on tiltboard. Arms and legs extended.

Test Stimulus

Tilt board to one side.

Negative Reaction

Head and thorax do not right themselves; no equilibrium or protective reactions. (It is possible to have positive reactions in some body parts but not in others.)

Positive Reaction

Righting of head and thorax, abduction and extension of arm and leg on raised side (equilibrium reaction), protective reaction on lowered side of board.

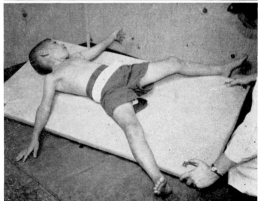

Positive Reaction

Positive reactions normal about six months of age and continue throughout life. Negative reaction after six months of age may be one indication of delayed reflexive maturation.

Prone

Negative Reaction

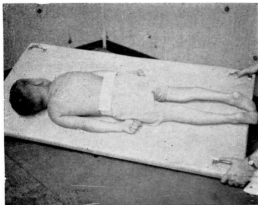

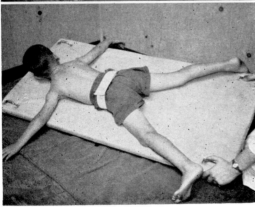

Positive Reaction

Test Position

Patient prone on tiltboard.
Arms and legs extended.

Test Stimulus

Tilt board to one side.

Negative Reaction

Head and thorax do not
right themselves; no
equilibrium or
protective reactions.
(It is possible to have
positive reactions in some
body parts but not in others.)

Positive Reaction

Righting of head and thorax,
abduction and extension of
arm and leg on raised side
(equilibrium reaction),
protective reaction on
lowered side of board.

Positive reactions normal about six months of age and continue throughout life. Negative reaction after six months of age may be one indication of delayed reflexive maturation.

Four-foot Kneeling

Negative Reaction

Test Position

Patient in quadruped position.

Test Stimulus

Tilt toward one side.

Negative Reaction

Head and thorax do not right themselves; no equilibrium or protective reactions.
(It is possible to have positive reactions in some body parts but not in others.)

Positive Reaction

Righting of head and thorax, abduction-extension of arm and leg on raised side (equilibrium reaction), and protective reactions on lowered side.

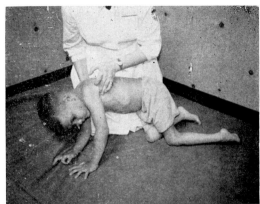

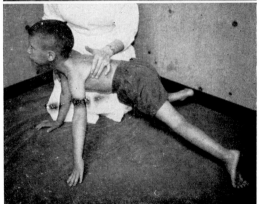

Positive Reaction

Positive reactions normal about eight months of age and continue throughout life. Negative reactions after eight months of age may be one indication of delayed reflexive maturation.

Sitting

Negative Reaction

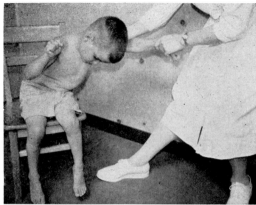

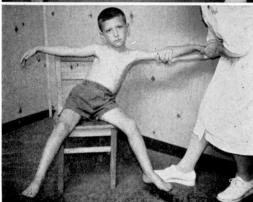

Positive Reaction

Test Position

Patient seated on chair.

Test Stimulus

Pull or tilt patient
to one side.

Negative Reaction

Head and thorax do not
right themselves; no
equilibrium or
protective reactions.
(It is possible to have positive
reactions in some body parts
but not in others.)

Positive Reaction

Righting of head and thorax,
abduction-extension of arm
and leg on raised side
(equilibrium reaction), and
protective reactions on
lowered side.

Positive reactions normal about ten to twelve months of age and continue throughout life. Negative reactions after twelve months of age may be one indication of delayed reflexive maturation.

Kneel-Standing

Negative Reaction

Test Position

Patient in kneel-standing position.

Test Stimulus

Pull or tilt patient to one side.

Negative Reaction

Head and thorax do not right themselves; no equilibrium or protective reactions. (It is possible to have positive reactions in some body parts but not in others.)

Positive Reaction

Righting of head and thorax, abduction-extension of arm and leg on raised side (equilibrium reaction), and protective reaction on lowered side of board.

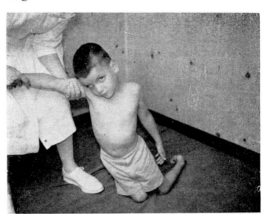

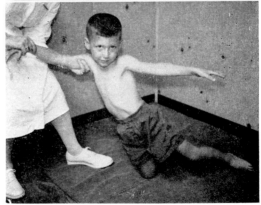

Positive Reaction

Positive reactions normal about fifteen months of age and continue throughout life. Negative reactions after fifteen months of age may be one indication of delayed reflexive maturation.

Negative Reaction   **Hopping 1**

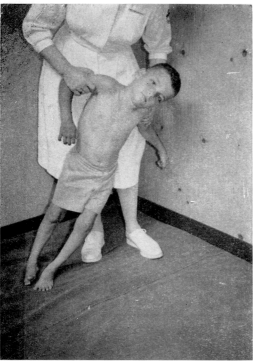

Test Position

Patient in standing position. Hold by upper arms.

Test Stimulus

Move to the left or to the right side.

Negative Reaction

Head and thorax do not right themselves; no hopping steps to maintain balance.

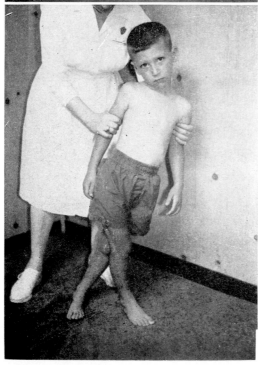

Positive Reaction

Righting of head and thorax, hopping steps sideways to maintain equilibrium.

Positive reactions normal about fifteen to eighteen months of age and continue throughout life. Negative reactions after eighteen months of age may be one indication of delayed reflexive maturation.

Positive Reaction

Hopping 2

Negative Reaction

Test Position

Patient in standing position. Hold by upper arms.

Test Stimulus

Move forward.

Negative Reaction

Head and thorax do not right themselves; no hopping steps to maintain balance.

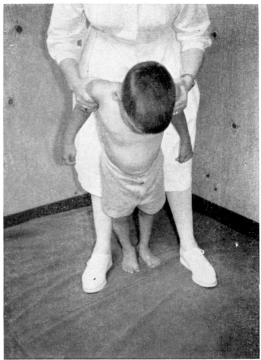

Positive Reaction

Righting of head and thorax, hopping steps forward to maintain equilibrium.

Positive reactions normal about fifteen to eighteen months of age and continue throughout life. Negative reactions after eighteen months of age may be one indication of delayed reflexive maturation.

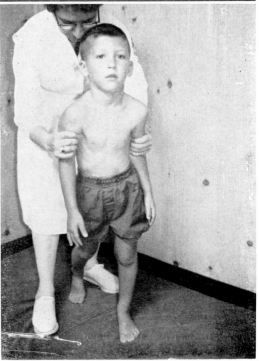

Positive Reaction

Negative Reaction　　　　　　　　　　　**Hopping 3**

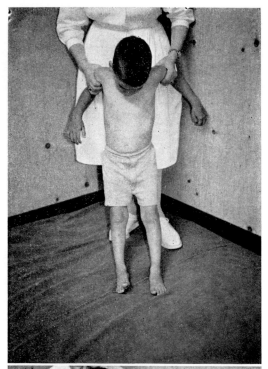

Test Position

Patient in standing position.
Hold by upper arms.

Test Stimulus

Move backwards.

Negative Reaction

Head and thorax do not right
themselves; no hopping steps
to maintain balance.

Positive Reaction

Righting of head and thorax,
hopping steps backwards
to maintain equilibrium.

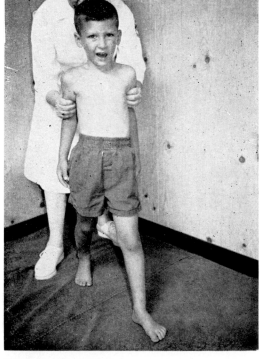

Positive reactions normal
about fifteen to eighteen
months of age and continue
throughout life. Negative reactions after eighteen months
of age may be one indication
of delayed reflexive maturation.

Positive Reaction

Dorsiflexion

Test Position

Patient in standing position. Hold under axillae.

Test Stimulus

Tilt patient backwards.

Negative Reaction

Head and thorax do not right thembselves; no dorsiflexion of feet.

Positive Reaction

Righting of head and thorax, feet dorsiflex.

Positive reactions normal about fifteen to eighteen months of age and continue throughout life. Negative reactions after eighteen months of age may be one indication of delayed reflexive maturation.

Negative Reaction

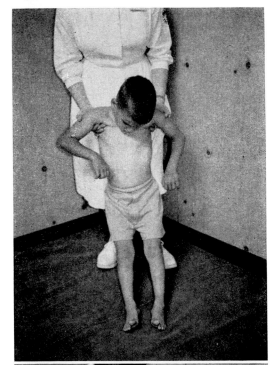

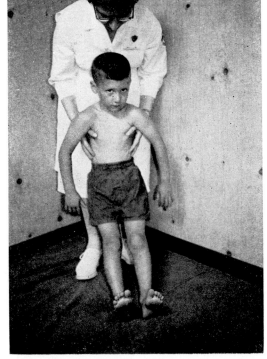

Positive Reaction

Negative Reaction

See-Saw

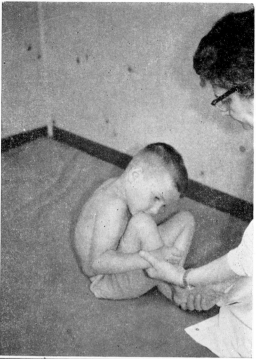

Test Position

(Patient must be able to maintain standing balance.) Patient in standing position. On same side, hold by hand and foot, flex hip and knee.

Test Stimulus

Pull arm forward gently and slightly to lateral side.

Negative Reaction

Head and thorax do not right themselves; Inability to maintain standing balance.

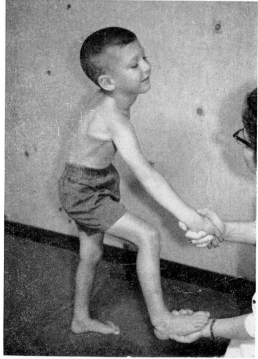

Positive Reaction

Righting of head and thorax, slight abduction and full extension of manually flexed knee to maintain equilibrium.

Positive reactions normal about fifteen months of age and continue throughout life. Negative reactions after fifteen months of age may be one indication of delayed reflexive maturation.

Positive Reaction

Simian Position

Test Position

Patient in squat-sitting position.

Test Stimulus

Tilt to one side.

Negative Reaction

Head and thorax do not right themselves; inability to assume or maintain position, lack of equilibrium or protective reactions.

Positive Reaction

Righting of head and thorax, abduction-extension of arm and leg on raised side (equilibrium reaction), and protective on the lowered side.

Negative Reaction

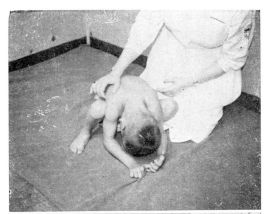

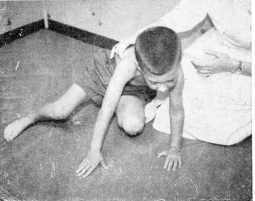

Positive Reaction

Positive reactions normal about fifteen to eighteen months of age and continue throughout life. Negative reactions after eighteen months of age may be one indication of delayed reflexive maturation.

NEWINGTON CHILDREN'S HOSPITAL

OCCUPATIONAL THERAPY DEPARTMENT

REFLEX TESTING CHART

Name: Reflex Level:

B.D.:   Therapist:

Date:

Reflexes	+	—	Comments:
1. Level One—Spinal:			
a. Flexor Withdrawal_____			_____
b. Extensor Thrust_____			_____
c. Crossed Extension_____			_____
2. Level Two—Brain Stem:			
a. Asymmetrical Tonic Neck____			_____
b. Symmetrical Tonic Neck_____			_____
c. Tonic Labyrinthine—supine___			_____
prone____			_____
d. Associated Reactions_____			_____
e. Positive Supporting Reaction___			_____
f. Negative Supporting Reaction__			_____
3. Level Three—Midbrain:			
Righting Reactions:			
a. Neck Righting_____			_____
b. Body Righting acting on the			
Body _____			_____
c. Labyrinthine Righting acting			
on the head_____			_____
d. Optical Righting_____			_____
e. Amphibian _____			
4. Automatic Movement Reactions:			
a. Moro Reflex_____			_____
b. Landau Reflex_____			_____
c. Protective Extensor Thrust____			_____
5. Level Four—Cortical:			
Equilibrium Reactions:			
a. Prone-lying _____			_____
b. Supine-lying _____			_____
c. Four-foot kneeling_____			_____
d. Sitting_____			_____
e. Kneel-standing _____			_____
f. Standing—hopping _____			_____
dorsiflexion _____			_____
see-saw_____			_____
g. Simian posture _____			_____

NEWINGTON CHILDREN'S HOSPITAL

OCCUPATIONAL THERAPY DEPARTMENT

MOTOR DEVELOPMENT CHART

Name: Date:

B.D.:   Dominance:

Reflex Level: Therapist:

Motor Development	*Comments:*

I. Head Raising:
   1. Prone (1-2 mos.): _____
   2. Supine (4-6 mos.): _____
   3. Sidelying (7 mos.): _____

II. Turning:
   1. Supine-sidelying (1-4 wks.): _____
   2. Supine-prone (6 mos.): _____
   3. Prone-supine (8 mos.): _____

III. Crawling (7-8 Mos.):
   1. Puppy dog: _____
   2. Static—makes amphibian movements: _____
   3. Creeps—makes amphibian movements;
      moves body forward: _____
   4. Bunnyhops—assumes 3 point crawling
      using complete rotation: _____
   5. Crawling—assumes 4 point crawling
      using complete rotation: _____
   6. Crawling—uses partial rotation up to sitting
      then assumes 4-foot kneeling and crawls: _____

IV. Sitting:
   1. Maintains (7 mos.): _____
   2. Assumes using complete rotation (10-12 mos.): _____
   3. Assumes using partial rotation (2-5 yrs.): _____
   4. Assumes symmetrically (5 yrs.): _____

V. Standing:
   1. Kneel-stands: _____
   2. Kneel-walks: _____
   3. Pulls up to standing (10½ mos.): _____
   4. Stands unassisted (14 mos.): _____
   5. Walks (15-18 mos.): _____

Continued →

Arm—Hand

Development	Comments:
0-4 mos. Reflexive grasp—no eye-hand coordination:_____	

4-8 mos. Conscious grasp—pronation:
    a. crude: _____
    b. between palmar and fingers—ulnar:_____
    c. thumb adducted, not utilized:_____	

6 mos. Eye-hand coordination begins:_____
    Arms used asymmetrically—control from
        shoulder and shoulder girdle:_____
    corralling reach:_____	

7 mos. Radial palmar grasp:_____	

8 mos. Scissor grasp:_____
    Thumb envelopes object:_____
    Elbow flexible:_____	

9 mos. Crude pinch—pincer grasp:_____
    Advertent release of grasp:_____
    Wrist flexibility:_____
    use of forearm between mid-position and
        pronation: _____	

11 mos. Pincer release:_____ Supination more frequently:_____	
12 mos. Opposition: _____ Supination—cortically controlled:_____	

CONCLUSION

T HE sequential development of normal and abnormal reflex maturation is presented with illustrations and techniques for testing and recording described. *Early evaluation* of abnormal reactions and the importance of *early referral* for treatment are stressed. It is hoped that this presentation will provide a clearer understanding and stimulate the use of a neurophysiologically-oriented approach in the evaluation, diagnosis and treatment of the child with cerebral dysfunction.

RECOMMENDED READING

Andre-Thomas: Integration in the infant. *Cerebral Palsy Bull., 8:3,* 1959.

Bobath, B.: Control of postures and movements in the treatment of cerebral palsy. *Physiotherapy, 39:99,* 1953.

Bobath, B.: The importance of the reduction of muscle tone and the control of mass reflex action in the treatment of spasticity. *Occup. Ther., 27:371,* 1948.

Bobath, B.: A new treatment of lesions of the upper motor neurone. *Br. J. Phys. Med., 2:26,* 1948.

Bobath, B.: A study of abnormal postural reflex activity in patients with lesions of the central nervous system, Parts 1-4. *Physiotherapy, 40:259, 295, 326, 368,* 1954.

Bobath, B.: The treatment of motor disorders of pyramidal and extra-pyramidal origin by reflex inhibition and by facilitation of movements. *Physiotherapy, 41:146,* 1955.

Bobath, K. and Bobath, B.: Spastic paralysis; treatment by the use of reflex inhibition. *Br. J. Phys. Med., 13:121,* 1950.

Bobath, K. and Bobath, B.: Tonic reflexes and righting reflexes in the diagnosis and assessment of cerebral palsy. *Cerebral Palsy Rev., 16* (5):4, 1955.

Bobath K. and Bobath, B.: A treatment of cerebral palsy based on the analysis of the patient's motor behavior. *Br. J. Phys. Med., 15:107,* 1952.

Bobath, K. and Bobath, B.: Control of motor function in the treatment of cerebral palsy. *Aust. J. Physiother, 2* (2):75, 1956.

Bobath, K. and Bobath. B.: Treatment of cerebral palsy by the inhibition of abnormal reflex action. *Br. Orthop. J., 11:1,* 1954.

Bobath, K.: The neuropathology of cerebral palsy and its importance in treatment and diagnosis. *Cerebral Palsy Bull., 8:13,* 1959.

Bobath, K. and Bobath, B.: An assessment of the motor handicap of children with cerebral palsy and of their response to treatment. *Occup. Ther. J.,* 1-16, 1958.

Bobath, B. and Finnie, N.: Re-education of movement patterns for everyday life in the treatment of cerebral palsy. *Occup. Ther. J.,* 1-8, 1958.

Bobath, B.: Observations on adult hemiplegia and suggestions for treatment. *Physiotherapy,* 1-23, 1959-1960.

Crickmay, M.: Description and Orientation of the Bobath Method with Reference to Speech Rehabilitation in Cerebral Palsy. Chicago, National Society of Crippled Children and Adults, 1956.

Fay, T.: Neurophysical aspects of therapy in cerebral palsy. *Arch. Phys. Med., 29:* 327, 1948.

Gesell, A. L., *et al.: The First Five Years of Life.* New York, Harper and Bros., 1940.

Henneman, E.: Spinal reflexes and the control of movement. In Mountcastle, V. M. (Ed.): *Medical Physiology.* St. Louis, Mosby, 1968, 12th ed., Vol. II, pp. 1733-1749.

Knoblock, H. and Pasamanick, B.: The developmental behavioral approach to the neurologic examination in infancy. *Child Dev., 33:*181, 1962.

Magnus, R.: Some results of studies in the physiology of posture. *Lancet, 2:*531, 1926.
Mysak, E. D.: Significance of neurophysiological orientation of cerebral palsy rehabilitation. *J. Speech Hear. Disord., 24* (3):221, 1959.
Mysak, E. D. and Fiorentino, M. R.: Neurophysiological consideration in occupational therapy for the cerebral palsied. *Am. J. Occup. Ther., 15* (3):113, 1961.

Paine, R. S.: Neurologic examination of infants and children. *Pediatr. Clin. North Am., 7* (3):471-510, 1960.
Paine, R. S.: The evolution of infantile postural reflexes in the presence of chronic brain syndromes. *Dev. Med. Child. Neurol., 6:*345-361, 1964.
Parmelee, A. H.: A critical evaluation of the Moro reflex. *Pediatrics, 33:*773-788, 1964.

Rood, M.: Neurophysiological reactions as a basis for physical therapy. *Phys. Ther. Rev., 34:*444, 1954.
Russell, W. R.: The physiology of memory. *Proc. R. Soc. Med., 51:*9, 1958.

Seamans, S.: A neurophysiological approach to treatment of cerebral palsy introduction to the Bobath method. *Phys. Ther. Rev., 38* (9):598.
Sherrington, C. S.: *Selected Writings.* (D. Denny-Brown, Ed.). London, Hamish Hamilton Medical Books, 1939.
Strauss, A. and Kephart, N. C.: *Psychopathology and Education of the Brain-Injured Child.* New York, Grune and Stratton, 1955, Vol. II.

Twitchell, T. E.: Sensory factors in purposive movement. *J. Neurophysiol., 17:*239, 1954.

Walshe, F. M.: On certain tonic or postural reflexes in hemiplegia with special reference to the so-called associated movements. *Brain, 46:*1, 1923.
Weisz, S.: Studies in equilibrium reaction. *J. Nerv. Ment. Dis., 88:*150, 1938.

INDEX